The
BUSINESS
Side of
DENTISTRY

The
BUSINESS
Side of
DENTISTRY

Philip L. Kempler D.M.D.

Bay City

PUBLISHING, LLC

Edited by Mikel Benton
Cover illustration by Michael Rohani
Book design by DesignForBooks.com

Printed in the U.S.A.

DISCLAIMER

Please Note: Information included in this book is
current at time of print and may not apply to your
particular situation. If you have questions regarding
your income taxes or Social Security benefits, please
contact your CPA or attorney.

Contents

Appendices

Overhead Analysis Templates

Retirement Analysis Templates

Preface

$\mathcal{W}$hen I bought my first practice in 1979 I didn't have a clue what to look for and there was no one to turn to for help. Oh sure, there were lots of brokers selling dental practices. But they were just sales people and they didn't know one type of dental practice from another. They understood how to complete the paper work but most, to be quite honest, cared more about the commission than helping a young dentist find a practice that was right for me. They never even asked what I was looking for as far as type of patient, type of procedures done in the office, whether I wanted a hygienist or wanted to do hygiene myself, how many patients I wanted to see each day, and lots of other questions that a knowledgeable broker would know to ask. Several years later, when I merged a small practice into my existing practice, I still had no one to turn to and the seller's broker was only interested in making a sale. Then, when I sold my first practice, a different broker, in order to get the listing, told me I could get a lot more money than my practice was actually worth. Once he had the listing all the offers that came in were substantially lower than the listing price. When I asked him why that was happening he said, "Maybe we have it listed too high." Then, the broker had the nerve to try to force me to sell. I felt like an idiot and I was totally frustrated.

It was about that time that I met Alan Thomas, Partner at *Thomas and Fees Accountancy Corporation,* an accounting firm that works almost exclusively with dentists. It was the first time I got answers to my questions from someone that understood the unique challenges of operating a dental business. "I better have the answers," Alan told me at our first visit, "I've been helping dentists develop their practices for over four decades."

It was Alan, in fact, that suggested I become a dental practice broker when I retired. "You'd be a terrific broker . . . you have unique insights into the practice purchase and sale experience. You know how to determine what a practice is worth and how to get it sold." But, what really motivated me was the idea that by becoming a dental practice broker, I could help my peers avoid the pitfalls I had endured. So, that's how it began some twenty five years ago.

The purchase or sale of your dental practice is one of the most important decisions of your life. You deserve an honest, trustworthy and knowledgeable representative that cares more about you than his or her commission.

Whatever phase of the industry you are in, whether you are looking for your first associate's position, buying your first practice or selling your practice and retiring, I wish you luck. I hope you find this information beneficial.

Sincerely,
Philip L. Kempler, D.M.D., Broker
Thomas & Fees Practice Sales

Part

1

Associate Compensation

1

What a Graduating Dentist can Expect in His or Her First Job

$\mathscr{C}$ongratulations. You made it through dental school and now it is time to get a real job. Let us assume that you are not starting your own practice from scratch (we will describe the disadvantages in doing so in the following chapter). The best option is to associate with an established dentist who either has too much work to handle alone or wants to start winding down. This is a great way to do real dentistry on real patients. While working as an associate in an existing practice, you will have time to increase your speed and you will learn how to manage your time. You will also begin to learn how a dental office really operates. In addition, you will have the benefit of an experienced dentist to consult with on a variety of matters including case presentation, office management, employee relations, and overhead.

How will you be paid during this period? Associate dentists can be paid a daily rate, a percentage, or a combination of both. A daily rate ranges between $500 to $1,000 per day, depending on the type of practice, the fee schedule, etc. A percentage is usually 25 or 30 percent of production. Some associates will make a base of $500 a day plus a percentage of anything over $2,000 per day of production. This often is the best way to go because initially you may not see many patients and the owner may want to take the big cases. If possible, try to get the owner to agree that you see new patients and get to perform all the treatment necessary. A written contract is a must. You want, in writing, an outline of your duties, responsibilities, compensation, and other pertinent conditions of employment.

With the increasing rise of "corporate dentistry" there is a second option available to recent grads. Corporate dentistry can be as small as one or more dentists who own several practices or as large as a corporation that owns hundreds of practices. These employers are always looking for dentists. The compensation may be on the lower end of the scale when compared to individual dentists, but the recent grad receives an opportunity to perform lots of dentistry and various procedures without having to worry about anything else, such as payments, insurance, etc. This allows you to increase your speed. If you should make an error, it is not on your patient. This gives you great experience in actually doing dentistry, which can be an invaluable tool should you decide to go into private practice. Corporate dentistry is not for everyone, but it is a viable alternative.

Lastly, the recent grad should be sure to have malpractice insurance in force before he or she ventures out into the real world. Nobody is infallible. Malpractice insurance is an important safeguard that you don't want to be without. Again, whichever route you choose, you should have a written contract listing you and your employer's responsibilities and duties. It's like poker: the more cards you have on the table, the better your hand.

In the following Chapter, a comparison of the three payment methods for new associates and the estimated take-home pay for each type of arrangement, as well as information on professional expenses.

How Will You be Compensated in Your Associate Job?

There are a number of different ways the employer could pay you. You could be an employee or an independent contractor. Your compensation could be based upon a salary per day, your production, or the amount ultimately collected (collections).

Here is how these methods affect your net pay. Let's assume that you produce $3,000 a day and the owner collects $2,750.

1 AS AN EMPLOYEE (w/2)		**1** AS AN INDEPENDENT CONTRACTOR (1099)	
Salary per day	750.00	Salary per day	750.00
Payroll taxes - Social Security - Disability	64.50	Self-employment tax	112.50
Income taxes - Estimated	225.00	Income taxes - Estimated	206.10
Take home	**$ 460.50**	**Take home**	**$ 431.40**

2	30% of production ($3,000 x 30%)	900.00		**2**	30% of production ($3,000 x 30%)	900.00
	Payroll taxes – Social Security – Disability	77.40			Self-employment tax	135.00
	Income taxes – Estimated	270.00			Income taxes – Estimated	249.90
	Take home	**$ 552.60**			**Take home**	**$ 515.10**
3	30% of collections ($2,750 x 30%)	825.00		**3**	30% of collections ($2,750 x 30%)	825.00
	Payroll taxes – Social Security – Disability	70.95			Self-employment tax	123.75
	Income taxes – Estimated	247.50			Income taxes – Estimated	228.90
	Take home	**$ 506.55**			**Take home**	**$472.35**

Professional expenses – Employee

As an employee your professional expenses are not deductible.

Professional expenses – Independent contractor

As an independent contractor, all professional expenses are able to be deducted.

What are professional expenses?

- ▶ Hand instruments acquired in dental school
- ▶ Library acquired in dental school
- ▶ Professional dues
- ▶ Continuing education, including travel, hotel, etc.
- ▶ Travel to second job location or lab
- ▶ Business meals
- ▶ Other directly related costs in performing your profession

Part

2

How to Buy a
Dental Practice

3

When Should You Buy?

*I*s it wise for a graduating dentist to buy a dental practice the minute he or she gets out of dental school? The answer is that it depends upon the dentist. Some dentists exit dental school with a working knowledge of how to run a business. Perhaps they took business courses in college or had experience working in family businesses prior to getting their diplomas. For those lucky few, the answer is yes. Because they are business savvy, buying a practice right out of school will probably work out just fine. For most new graduates, however, it is rarely a good idea.

Taking a job as an associate dentist for several years allows you to gain experience in the dental field and familiarize yourself with the business side of dentistry. It allows you to make mistakes on the other doctor's dime, and if the dentist you are working with is highly successful, you can learn proven techniques for everything from how to handle employees to patient scheduling. The knowledge you can gain from a position in a thriving practice is invaluable.

Also, if you're happy in your first position and stay a while, you may be able to purchase the practice from the owner when he or she retires. Wouldn't it be great to purchase a practice where you understand staff dynamics, you're familiar with the patient base, and have realistic business expectations about the value of the practice?

One last point: Working as an associate for two or three years gives you time to discover the kind of practice you want in your future. You may graduate from dental school thinking that you want to practice one kind of dentistry and discover that you enjoy something totally different. Experience is a great teacher.

CASE STUDY **1**

Saved by the bell

I remember the day I graduated from dental school. I was so sure of myself and my dental skills. I was ready to take on the world. There was only one problem: I didn't have a clue how to run a business. Oh sure, I had worked for my dad in the summers at his building supply company, but I drove a truck.

Yes we had talked business over dinner, so I knew more than most about handling overhead and keeping costs in line. Plus, because I was a math whiz, working with numbers and overhead came easy to me. But the truth was that I had never hired or fired an employee. I had never had to make a payroll or deal with insurance companies. My interaction with people was in a controlled environment with little personal risk. If I did something wrong or needed advice on how to handle a situation someone more experienced was always nearby.

Thankfully, I took advice from an older peer and started taking classes about business and, specifically, about how to run a dental practice. Those classes made me realize that there were a lot of things I didn't know how to do, like patient scheduling, case presentation, hygiene department development, and collections. Getting assistance from an older, more experienced dentist was a real eye-opener and saved me time, money, and grief when I started my own practice. As the saying goes, I was saved by the bell.

4

Where Should You Buy Your Practice?

When a dentist contacts me and says, "I want to buy a dental practice," I always ask, "What are you looking for?" If the dentist replies that he is "flexible," I know that he needs to give the question more thought. I can't tell you how many practices I've had to sell for dentists who, in a relatively short period of time, had become "sick and tired of commuting an hour back and forth to work."

Look for a practice within thirty minutes of your home or the city you plan to live in. Close proximity to your practice is beneficial for four reasons:

Emergency patients can be great practice builders, as long as your office is not so far from home that emergencies are more of a hassle than an asset.

Being close to your office reduces daily stress, gives you more time with your family, and makes it easy to do paperwork in the evenings, if need be.

Automobile costs are greatly reduced when you work and live close to home.

When you live close to where you work, you have the opportunity to become a visible entity in the community. Becoming part of the community helps you make connections with parents of your children, teachers, neighbors, and other businessmen. Connections in the community create visibility and can be a driver of patients into the practice.

Obviously there are other considerations when purchasing a practice, such as the visibility of the location, accessibility to roads and freeways, size of active patient base in the area, and plans for future growth in the area. All of these considerations should be explored.

CASE STUDY **2**

It seemed like a good idea at first

I remember speaking to a dentist who had purchased a practice an hour and a half from home. We were at the dental convention and he stopped at our booth to inquire about listing the practice for sale. "You know," he said, "I honestly thought three hours a day on the road would help me clear my mind. And I thought I could use the time to learn another language or something. But in reality, the long drive became a total drag."

This dentist wasn't the first one to tell that story. We had another dentist who thought he could handle driving to Los Angeles from Orange County every day. We helped the dentist sell that practice and buy another just a few blocks from his home. A month or so after the sale, he called and said, "Dr. Kempler, selling that practice was the best decision I ever made. Thanks a million. You gave me back my life."

Chapter

5

How much is the practice worth?

$\mathcal{T}$here are many methods for valuing dental practices. Most experts favor the income-based approach. The income-based approach recognizes the critical components of a successful practice: practice income, expenses, and appropriate compensation for the owner. Owner compensation is not just the amount listed on your tax return. Total compensation includes additional items such as the value of health insurance, company car, trips, and patient entertainment. And even though the IRS may deem these so-called perks to be taxable income, the income listed on a tax return or a profit and loss statement is not necessarily the same amount of income that was earned by the seller or could be earned by the buyer.

Buying a practice is not like buying a house. When you buy a house you base your decision on the monthly payment you can afford. That's not how it works when purchasing a practice. Don't get fixated on a maximum or minimum purchase price of say $200,000. Find the practice that suits you best and, once you find it, ask the broker to show you how the price was determined. Don't be afraid to spend $800,000 or even $1,000,000 to buy the *right* practice, as long as you feel confident enough to handle the estimated daily production and there is sufficient cash flow to service the debt and provide you with good take-home pay. An experienced broker, or good dental accountant, will be able to help you make that determination.

CASE STUDY 3

Case presentations patients will accept

"I only want to spend between $150,000 and $200,000 for a practice. That's my limit. Period!" That was how my conversation began with a young dentist from Riverside.

"Ok," I said. "Why is that the maximum price?"

He answered simply, "I don't want to get in over my head."

While I totally appreciated that this young dentist was trying to make a responsible financial decision about his future, I realized that he didn't understand that purchasing a lower-priced practice didn't guarantee financial success. A failing $150,000 practice wasn't any better than a failing $400,000 practice. If this young dentist wanted a secure financial future, he needed to find a thriving practice with a patient base that wanted the kind of dentistry he enjoyed doing. He needed to look at the total picture. Fixating on the price alone was not the answer. After a discussion of cash flow, he understood that the price was only one part of the puzzle. He needed to look at the total business. The income, overhead, and patient charts needed to be analyzed. He did his due diligence and we found him a $400,000 practice in Riverside, where he lived, that could support the debt and give him excellent take-home pay. His decision was sound and met his criteria for a secure financial future.

6

Practice Preferences – What Kind of Practice Should You Buy?

The kind of practice you want to buy will depend upon the kind of dentistry you want to do. Choose a practice that fits your dental expertise and temperament. For example, if you enjoy a slower-paced environment and want to see only a few patients a day, you'd be miserable in a practice that sees twenty or more patients a day. Likewise, if you enjoy a fast-paced environment, you wouldn't be happy in a small practice. Also, you should consider the patient makeup of the practice.

If the typical patient is in a lower socioeconomic class and only wants "necessary" dentistry performed, be sure that's okay with you. On the other hand, if you want to do ideal dentistry and have a high acceptance rate of your treatment plans, you will want a practice that supports that kind of dentistry. Likewise, if the majority of the patients are of a particular ethnic group, make sure that is acceptable to you. This may sound obvious, but I see it all the time. Doing the kind of dentistry you enjoy is what makes being a dentist fun.

CASE STUDY 4

Case presentations patients will accept

"Help me find a different practice!" That was the plea I received one day on my answering machine. When I spoke to the dentist who had left the message, he told me that when he got out of dental school he hadn't really given the location of his practice enough thought. "I bought the first practice I could find in my hometown. I want to do cosmetic dentistry and I thought I could convince my patients to want it too. But these nice folks just don't have the finances to accept the cases I present. All I do is drill and fill. I'm miserable."

This was a good practice, but it was not a good practice for **this** dentist. He made the mistake of thinking that the only reason the prior dentist hadn't done cosmetic dentistry was because he hadn't been presenting it properly. He thought that with his dynamic case presentation skills he could gain case acceptance and make an excellent income doing the type of dentistry he loved. It didn't take him long to realize that not every patient can afford cosmetic dentistry, no matter how well it is presented or how wonderful it makes your smile.

We got his practice sold and he moved his family to Irvine, California, a city with patients who want and can afford cosmetic dentistry. When I last spoke to him, the doctor said, "Life is good, Dr. Kempler. You should see the beautiful smiles I'm making. Thanks!"

7

Buy Versus Build

W hen you start the quest to open your own practice, it's natural to wonder if it would be better to buy an existing practice or start your own from scratch. I've heard practitioners say, "I can build a practice for a lot less money than the practices I find on the market." While that's probably true, in the long run buying an existing practice is less pricey and less risky as well. Let me explain why:

> When you purchase an existing practice, you purchase an operational dental business with an immediate patient base and dependable revenue stream.

> It takes three times as much money to bring new patients into your practice as it does to generate income from an established patient base. Therefore, while the price tag of an existing practice can be higher than the out-of-pocket costs of a startup, the practice purchase is usually less costly overall.

The return on investment (ROI) is faster when you purchase an existing practice. When you start from scratch, it takes time after the practice is operational to advertise, promote a new practice, and entice patients through your front door. And it takes time and money to diagnose treatment, deliver that treatment, and collect from patients and insurance companies. Your overhead costs start immediately but your cash flow does not. With an existing practice, ROI (money back in the bank) begins immediately upon close of escrow. As I said before, when you start a practice from scratch, ROI takes time.

Financing an ongoing business is easier than financing a start-up. Banks consider a start-up a higher risk than a proven commodity like an existing practice. And where there is higher risk, there is higher cost.

Finally, it takes lots of time and energy to build a practice. There are hundreds of decisions to make. You'll have to find, interview, and hire employees. You will need to negotiate insurance contracts and make equipment purchases. The research required for each of these decisions will be time consuming and intensive. With an existing practice, all those hassles, decisions, and purchases—and the accompanying stress—have been dealt with, leaving you free to practice dentistry.

CASE STUDY **5**

The practice of my dreams

When I first met Dr. G., she was in the middle of building her Taj Mahal of a practice in the desert. She was so excited and thrilled. "It's the practice of my dreams," she told me with a smile that covered her face. A few months later we met at the dental convention. Dr. G. was in another state of mind. She was exhausted, strung out, and totally frustrated. "I'm spending so much more money than I thought I would. New equipment costs are killing me. This project is consuming my life. I hope all this work will be worth it in the end."

I wished Dr. G. well as she wandered away from our booth, and I meant it. I hoped that she'd come through the building experience happy and whole, but I didn't envy her position. Building a practice from scratch is not an experience for the faint of heart.

I had no doubt it would be a beautiful facility. But, I know from twenty-five years of experience buying and selling dental practices that Dr. G. had a long, hard road ahead. The building was almost done but a reliable revenue stream was still nowhere in sight. As I have said before, in most cases buying an existing practice is a much better decision than starting one from scratch.

8

It's Time for Due Diligence

*O*k, let's say that you have found the right type of practice, in the right location, and you have agreed upon the price. Now, it's time for due diligence.

Due diligence is when you find out if what the seller has told you about the practice is true. In the buy/sell agreement you will be allotted a certain number of days for due diligence (normally ten days from the time your offer is accepted). The seller will not allow the practice to be reserved for an indefinite period of time in case the buyer decides against the purchase. In order to complete the task, you must have unobstructed access to the following:

- The practice.
- Three years of tax returns and financial statements, including the most recent operating income statement.
- Bank statements, two or three years' worth.
- Production report by procedure.

- The appointment book.

- An inventory of all the equipment and furniture being sold with the practice.

- Employee information including salaries, number of days worked, benefits, and length of service with the practice.

- Accounts receivable with aging summary.

- Fee schedule.

- Access to all patient records.

- Information on all insurance plans the practice contracted with.

- Office lease agreement with addenda for the practice

All of the above items will need to be methodically audited prior to completion of the sale. However, many should have been discussed and revealed *prior* to the due diligence period. The audit should be conducted in a step-by-step manner so that nothing is missed. The seller should be available to answer questions during the process.

1. MOST IMPORTANT – **Auditing collections.** Collections will show up on computer production reports, tax returns, and financial statements. Audit the collections to verify that the amount of collections presented to the buyer are verified by the bank statements.

2. **Auditing of financial records.** Unless your broker is highly knowledgeable in the dental field, I strongly recommend that you get help from a specialist (a dental accountant or CPA). Obviously, it would be a conflict of interest to allow the seller's broker to review the financial records.

3. **Auditing patient records.** Determine the number of active patient charts that are in the files. (Active patients in this instance is defined as different patients seen in the last year.) Choose a number of patient charts to examine. I recommend twenty-five to thirty. Compare the treatment plans with the x-rays and the progress notes with the treatments. See if the treatment was actually billed to the insurance company or the patient. See if the type of dentistry delivered was something you would likely provide. Check the financial arrangements on the charts. Check the progress notes for accuracy and completeness. Check the schedule to see if the patient actually came in as noted in the charts.

Most importantly, check to see if the dentist has undiagnosed treatments left in the charts that you would normally diagnose. And see if the dentist has over-treated or over-diagnosed treatments in the charts that you would not normally choose to do.

4. **Auditing patient scheduling.** Examine patient scheduling, both past and current. Determine if the practice uses a scheduling system or appoints haphazardly. See how hygiene appointments are handled. Determine how many new patients the practice is getting each month. Also, see how much time is allotted for procedures. Does the time allotment match up with the amount of time it takes you to complete that particular procedure?

5. **Audit employee records.** Check wages, salaries, benefits, time in service, and relationship to seller, if any. A good broker should provide you with all that information from day one. It's important information and part of the practice puzzle.

CASE STUDY **6**

Buyer beware

We had a doctor in central Orange County who had gone to school with the seller's brother. Because of that fact, the buyer said, "I know the family and I trust him. I don't need to go through the charts." The buyer did examine the tax returns. Despite numerous discussions on the phone and my pleading to consult with an expert and complete his due diligence, the doctor ignored my recommendations. He wanted the practice closed as quickly as possible. Once the buyer took possession of the practice, he quickly discovered that the seller had been billing insurance companies for procedures not performed.

He had put sealants on teeth that had not erupted in the mouth. He had billed insurance for sealants on teeth that already had sealants placed on them. And he billed for two-surface fillings when only one surface was involved. The practice was rampant with fraudulent billing. The case went to court and both parties suffered greatly in time and money.

9

From Buyer to Boss:
What Needs to be Done?

*W*hen you take over the dental practice, you not only take responsibility of the patients, you start a relationship with the staff. As buyer you become the employer. A practice sale can trigger a bevy of emotions for you and staff members alike. In addition, you have legal obligations to your new employees that must be dealt with correctly to prevent potential violations of federal employment laws. Both buyer and seller must be protected during the transition period.

Some dentists are under the illusion that federal laws don't apply to them because they have very few employees. This is not the case. Federal employment laws apply to all businesses, regardless of size.

Let's look at how federal employment laws might affect transitioning staff and the principal parties of the sale. Let's say that the seller had several employees who have been with the practice for varying periods of time. And let's assume that the employees want to keep their positions after the sale, which is the case 99 percent of the time. Employees generally want and need the jobs. If the seller fails to terminate the staff members officially with written notices and fails to get proofs or receipts of those notices, the seller could be liable for any errors the new employer (the buyer) makes.

For example, let's say that the buyer doesn't pay a staff member adequately for overtime. Without proper documentation of termination, the seller could be liable for the overtime pay along with any penalties and interest the labor board assesses.

Even worse, the labor board can review all documents pertaining to the case, as well as those of other employees, and their investigation can go back three years. The buyer, even though he had nothing to do with the employees prior to purchasing the practice, could be liable for any violations made by the seller in the past along with penalties and interest. The amounts owed could be enormous. As you can see, both parties need to be protected during the practice sale.

In order to protect the buyer and the seller, both parties must take action. The buyer must interview each employee and rehire him or her individually (as an employee at will, of course). The seller must terminate each employee in writing and with proof of receipt. These two actions break the chain of employment and help protect both parties from employee law claims arising from the actions of their counterparts.

One last point about handling the employees: We live in a litigious society, especially here in California. Your employees are being educated by attorneys on TV to "know their employee rights." They are being encouraged to take their employers to court if their federally mandated rights have been violated. You can't depend on ignorance of the labor laws to protect you. Your employees are getting smarter by the day. And, trust me, there are employees out there who wouldn't hesitate to take their bosses to court if they felt they had suffered harm. This is another reason to work with an experienced and knowledgeable practice broker.

The letter you send to the patients

Once the sale of the practice has been finalized, and the staff has been informed, a letter is sent out to all current, active patients. The letter I have used for years has been very well received. It thanks the patients for all their years of trust and introduces the new dentist and his or her qualifications. Both buyer and seller review the letter *before* it is printed on the seller's stationery, signed by the seller, and mailed.

CASE STUDY 7

My employees would never do that!

I am no longer amazed by how seemingly wonderful and devoted employees can quickly turn on their boss when money is involved. So I wasn't surprised when Dr. R. called me and said, "Dr. Kempler, you're not going to believe this. My chairside assistant took me to the labor board. She says I owe her overtime and she didn't get her breaks. The labor board says I owe her $8,000 in back pay and overtime." Dr. R, like many in the industry, thought of his employees as friends. He didn't believe a time clock was needed and, like too many dentists, he didn't have detailed time records. The labor board *always* decides for the employee when that is the case.

10

Tax Consequences of Buying a Practice

*T*here can be substantial tax consequences for both parties in the sale of a dental practice. In general terms, the assets being sold in a dental practice include equipment, patient records, dental supplies, furniture, fixtures, goodwill, and the covenant not to compete. The tax consequences have to do with how the various assets are allocated in the sale price. By changing the allocation value of the various assets, you can change the amount of tax that is owed. Simply put, the seller's objective is usually to allocate the sale price of the assets to minimize the income tax owed on the gain. The buyer, on the other hand, would like to allocate the purchase price to accelerate the tax deduction on the assets. How the allocation is negotiated can have a significant bearing on the agreed-upon price.

This is where a broker can really help. His negotiation skills, experience, and knowledge can make or break a deal. A conscientious, experienced, and principled broker will ensure that the purchase and sale of a dental practice is structured so that the process is a win-win situation for all concerned. Obviously, you'll want to meet with your CPA and attorney in *advance* of signing any documents to ensure that you are properly protected in the transaction. The importance of planning ahead cannot be overstated.

CASE STUDY 8

Penny wise and pound foolish

I think it was my dad who said, "The trick to life is knowing what you don't know." And when it comes to taxes and the IRS, not knowing what you don't know can be detrimental to your financial health. I remember hearing a guy talking one night at a CDA fundraiser. He was telling his buddies that he was buying a practice from the dentist he worked for and, "We're saving a bundle by not using a broker, attorney, or CPA." When one of the listeners asked him how he knew what to do, he answered confidently, "It's easy. We just copied his old contract and wrote it up ourselves."

Maybe everything turned out just fine for that dentist and his friend. I hope so, for their sake. But I doubt it. The world and especially the tax laws have changed in the last thirty years. Not getting advice from experts on matters as crucial as taxes and the purchase and sale agreement can make the broker's fee look like a pittance. Dentists are smart folks, but their expertise is in dentistry, not business. Things turn out better for people who know what they don't know and get help to fill in the knowledge gaps.

11

How to Choose a Practice Broker

𝒩 o two dentists are alike, and so too with dental brokers. When choosing a dental practice broker, look for experience, integrity, and proven expertise in the industry. Most dental practice brokers hire salespeople to answer the phones. This can be frustrating and a colossal waste of time, having to explain the same stuff to a different person each time you call the broker's office. Ask with whom you'll be speaking when you call the office. And if your contact person changes with the weather, find another broker. Look for a broker with banking contacts, dental attorney contacts, and CPA connections. Be sure your broker has a working knowledge of how a dental office operates and understands the difference between a fee-for-service office and managed care office. It's critically important to buy a practice that not only fits your needs, but fits your skills and temperament as well. When you buy the right practice, you not only enjoy dentistry more but you set yourself on the path to a successful dental career.

A retired dentist makes a better broker

I believe being a dentist gives me special insights that a non-dentist broker doesn't have. Most brokers aren't dentists. They don't know the difference between one practice and another. Being a dentist, I do. Because I'm a dentist, I understand how to read patient charts. Oftentimes I can see incomplete dentistry in those charts that a new dentist might be able to tap. Or I see in the charts that the selling doctor has very little dentistry left to be completed. Being able to read patient charts is an asset that non-dental brokers lack.

Also, I understand overhead and know what the norms should be. Practice numbers tell a story if the reader knows the language. Because I practiced dentistry for over fifteen years, I'm savvy to what the numbers say. This is really helpful when matching buyers and sellers. And it's incredibly important when dealing with banks who will loan money to the buyers.

I know how new patient flow fits into the picture as well. And in-depth knowledge of practice management can be a powerful negotiating tool. Plus, my dental experience helps me see and understand the *kind* of practice I am trying to sell. Knowing whether the buyer is a good fit for the practice I have listed can be extremely beneficial. For example, if the buyer wants a low-key practice seeing only a few patients a day, a face-paced managed care facility would be an unlikely fit.

In short, as a retired dentist, I know the important questions to ask. And I know what the answers to those questions say about the practice I am selling. For example: What kind of procedures does the seller do? Does he do endo? Does he place implants? Does he do ortho? Does he do his own hygiene or does he have a hygienist? And, as I've said before, how many patients a day does he see? These are essential considerations when trying to match a buyer and seller.

CASE STUDY **9**

Why I became a practice broker

The reason I became a practice sales broker was because of my desire to help my peers. And the reason I thought my fellow dentists needed help was because of the experiences I had when selling my practice. When I sold my practice in 1992, I interviewed two different brokers, both of whom were well known. They both told me I could get a very high selling price, higher than I expected. Alan Thomas, my accountant, warned me that he didn't think that price was reasonable. But I fell for the bait. I should have listed to Alan.

Months passed without an offer, and, finally, when I started getting offers they were significantly lower than the listing. Not a few thousand less, but tens of thousands less. The broker I had picked told me that I should take the offer and that he couldn't guarantee the price we had agreed upon. I felt betrayed and lied to. The broker made me feel like an idiot, like my best interests were not being considered. He wanted his commission.

That experience influences how we treat our clients. Today, when I take a listing, I *put in writing* that if I can't get the price at which I appraised the practice, then the seller has no obligation whatsoever to accept the offer. The choice is solely the seller's. I never force anyone to sell. And I never make a seller feel like an idiot. I try very hard to educate the seller before taking the listing and during the entire process.

Part

3

Sale of Your Practice and Retirement

12

Is it Really Time to Sell?

"Why do you want to sell your practice?"

$\mathcal{T}$hat's the first question I ask when I meet with a prospective client. It's important because many times the client is not selling for the right reason. Selling the practice is a permanent solution, while the reason the doctor is selling may be temporary. Maybe the dentist is just burned out or is experiencing personal issues or stress that can be resolved. And if the problems could be resolved, selling the practice would be a total mistake. A good broker will help a prospective client explore alternatives, like bringing in an associate or cutting back the hours worked, before taking a listing on the practice.

On the other hand, there are reasons why it might be the right time to sell the practice. Perhaps you have a physical or mental impairment that is preventing the delivery of dental care. Or perhaps you have the financial ability to retire and want freedom to explore other interests.

Knowing why you want to sell your practice and whether you are financially prepared to quit are two elements that must be considered thoroughly. Otherwise, you might make a decision that you regret.

CASE STUDY 10

Right move or wrong decision?

"I'm out of here. I want to get rid of this practice and I want to sell it fast!" When I hear something like that from a prospective seller, I know that there is more going on than just selling a dental practice. Dr. L. left a message like that on my answering service. When I called him back, he explained that he was getting a divorce and he just couldn't keep his mind on work. "My mind is all over the place," he explained frantically. "Just come and list my darn practice. I can't take it anymore."

Later that afternoon, after all the employees had gone home for the day, Dr. L. and I sat down for a good long talk. He had a beautiful practice in La Jolla, California. I am sure it was the envy of every other dentist in town. Dr. L. loved his patients and he loved the kind of dentistry that living in La Jolla provided him. I knew it would be an easy practice to sell, but selling is not what Dr. L. needed.

In the past twenty-five-plus years of working as a practice sales broker, I've come to know that selling under stress is never smart. It is a permanent solution to a transitional problem. Instead, I suggested that he cut back to a few days a week and bring in an associate. That would give him some breathing room to handle his stress. I suggested that he find someone he could talk to about what was happening in his life. Change can be very difficult to handle, especially divorce. Getting help can be the answer.

I felt relieved when Dr. L. agreed to take my suggestion. He hired a part-time associate and began to work on his emotional state. It didn't take long for him to begin to feel better. Six months later he left another message on my cell phone. "Hi, Dr. Kempler. I just wanted you to know that I am beginning to feel better about my life. The divorce is still happening, but I've come to realize it's not the end of my life or my dental career. Thanks for helping me put it all into the right perspective."

13

How Much is Your Practice Worth?

*D*etermining the value of a dental practice doesn't change whether you're the buyer or the seller. In both cases the overhead affects practice value and your take-home pay. Therefore, the material that follows is copied verbatim from Part 2 of this book.

Let me show you again how overhead affects practice value. Let's say that you gross $500,000 annually. That's above average for many dental practices. And let's say that your overhead is 78 percent, or $390,000. In this scenario, your net would be $110,000 and the value of your practice would be approximately $200,000. That's okay, but not great.

On the other hand, let's say you grossed the same $500,000 and kept your overhead to 63 percent, or $315.000. In this scenario, your net jumps to $185,000 and the value of your practice increases to approximately $370,000. That's a huge difference, and we see that all the time. Also, the $75,000 difference in net between the two practices is for only one year. After ten years you've lost three-quarters of a million dollars in profit, and that's for the same number of days worked and the very same workload. (These values do not include the accounts receivable.)

In short, if you want to get the value of your practice to increase, reduce your overhead. It's not a huge gross that will impress a buyer; it is a huge net.

CASE STUDY **11**

You can't pick a number out of the air

Last year, I met with a dentist who wanted to sell his practice. He had listed it with another broker the year before, but it never sold. When I asked him why, he said that there were two offers but they were way too low. Upon further discussion, he mentioned that the listing price was $450,000 and one offer was for $375,000 and the other was $365,000. His broker had told him that they could get $450,000 easily. I asked to look at his tax returns and profit and loss statements, and did a quick evaluation. The real value of the practice was around $375,000.

He reiterated what his broker had told him. Needless to say, he was not a happy camper when I showed him how practices are really appraised, using numbers and proven formulas. Many buyers today will hire either a dental accountant or a dental broker to appraise the value of a potential office prior to making an offer. Since the two offers he received were right on target of the true value, it was likely that both buyers had appraisals done by experts in the field. I suggested that the doctor think about what we had discussed and call me if he had any questions. About two weeks later, he called me and I listed the practice. Three months after I took the listing, the practice sold for $370,000.

Preparing the
Practice for Sale

A common question dentists ask when considering selling their practice is whether they should paint and re-carpet prior to sale. Ordinarily, the answer is no, unless the practice is in really bad repair. Obviously, you want to make sure that the office is clean and uncluttered, and that everything is in good working order. But you have to remember that the buyer might not like the color of the new carpet and want to change it. Also, it is not wise to buy new equipment just prior to sale. Buyers will rarely pay the full price for the equipment you purchase, regardless of the condition.

CASE STUDY **12**

No bang for your buck

Several years ago, a dentist from Torrance, California, contacted me about selling his practice. When I asked him why, he said that he was tired, had plenty of money to retire, and was seventy-four years old. I scheduled a meeting at his office after hours. The office was neat, had beautiful marble floors in the waiting room and the hallways to the operatories, and the wallpaper looked new. He had four operatories, and the equipment in two of the operatories was on the old side, but two ops had what looked like new equipment.

I asked him about those two ops, and he told me that he had been thinking about selling for a while and thought if he fixed up the office it would be easier to sell. He was worried that the production had gradually decreased over the last several years and thought that if the office looked newer, he could get a better sale price. Not only did he buy new equipment, he tore up the carpet in the waiting room and hallway and put in marble. On top of that, he put new wallpaper in the waiting room. He thought it really "spiffed up the joint" (his words, not mine).

When I returned to my office, I did a thorough appraisal, factoring in the collection figures after reviewing his tax returns and financial statements, using three mathematical appraisal methods. He was a little disappointed with the result. He said, "I just spent over $20,000 to remodel the office. Doesn't that count?" Unfortunately, it doesn't. Once I showed him the numbers, he agreed to list the practice at a fair price.

It didn't take long before I had a very interested party. I checked the buyer's credit and a visit with the dentist was arranged. They liked each other and an offer was made and accepted. The buyer and my seller met another time when the buyer visited the office to review the charts during his due diligence period. All was going great. The buyer asked if he could bring in his wife, and my seller agreed. Little did we know that the buyer's wife was an interior decorator. She hated the marble floors and thought they made the office look "too cold." She insisted that the floors would have to be torn out and replaced with wood floors.

She said the wallpaper was "hideous" (again, her words, not mine). They wanted a $15,000 credit to remodel. My seller was beside himself. He had just spent $20,000 and thought the place looked great. He was adamant that he was not going to "lose" another $15,000. Even herculean efforts on my part couldn't get either buyer or seller to budge, and the deal didn't go through. The moral of the story is talk to your broker **before** you want to sell to determine what, if any, improvements need to be made prior to listing your practice. As they say, "Beauty is in the eye of the beholder."

Your Behavior During the Sale and Why You Should not Tell the Staff

*W*henever I take a listing, I explain to the doctor that during the listing period he should continue to manage the practice as he has done in the past. Reducing his hours, days worked weekly, or cutting back on effort can negatively affect income and, thereby, the value of the practice. If the income declines, the bank and a potential buyer may not believe that the initial asking price of the practice is fair.

For many dentists the value of the practice is less of a concern than how they will handle the staff. Staff members in a dental office are extremely close. I've heard many a dentist say, "My staff members are not like employees; they are like family and friends." Because of this, many dentists want to tell the staff that they are putting the practice up for sale. They want to be upfront and honest. While I respect their reasoning, we don't recommend the staff be made aware of the pending sale. Here are the reasons why:

First, in 98 percent of the practices we sell, staff members are not told of the sale. The reason that number is high is because experience has proven that telling the staff about the sale can be detrimental to the sale. Second, knowledge of the potential sale cannot benefit the seller or the buyer.

Staff may tell patients and interfere with the transition from one doctor to the next. Or worse, patients hearing about the sale may seek out new dentists. Also, staff may flee the practice in search of other jobs, leaving the seller and the buyer in the lurch. Your goal during the listing period should be to have the practice continue without interruption so that the income revenue remains constant. Once staff knows, suppliers may find out and spread the word that you are selling. The dental industry, as you well know, is very tightly knit. When the general public knows of a pending sale, nothing good can come from it. That's one of the reasons we give sellers our evening phone number. We don't want sellers talking in the office about potential sales.

One last point: While the practice is being sold, we do everything possible to minimize the amount of time the dentist needs to take away from practicing dentistry. We do this because it's our job. More importantly, we do it because we want to ensure that the business maintains its normal cash flow. Remember, dentistry is your full-time job. Selling dental practices is mine.

CASE STUDY **13**

Me and my big mouth

"Dr. Kempler, my hygienist quit today. I can't get a temp immediately. I have a packed schedule these next three weeks, and her departure is going to cost me a fortune!"

I have to say, honestly, I was irritated when I got the call. It wasn't like I hadn't warned him to keep his listing a secret. He knew full well not to tell a soul. But, like many dentists, he believed his employees were like family and could be trusted completely. His hygienist was not a bad person. She was truly sorry to "jump ship," as he described it, but she had heard gossip that the buying doctor was difficult to work for. She wasn't going to take any chances with her employment.

An opening came up with a dentist much closer to her home, and she jumped at the chance to be in his employment. That's what can happen when the word gets out that the practice is being sold. Not only that, but she had a loyal following of hygiene patients and the doctor was concerned he'd lose more than a few. The moral to this story goes back to World War II: "Loose lips sink ships!"

16

Emotional Aspects of Selling Your Practice

*L*et's assume that the reasons are right and it's time to sell your practice. Hopefully, you've found an excellent broker to assist you in the sale. If the broker does his job, the sale should go smoothly and you and the broker will be working as partners. Your broker should prepare you for what to expect. However, even the best broker can't prepare you for the emotional aspects of the sale. Let's divide the emotional aspects into three different categories.

First and foremost is the reaction of the staff to the sale. As I've said before, if you're like most dentists, your staff is like family. If they are kept out of the negotiations and are left in the dark about the sale (which happens 98 percent of the time), it can be quite a shock. We have seen employees openly weep. Unlike many typical businesses, the dentist often has a close relationship with staff members and may consider them his or her best friends. After working all day with the same faces four or five days a week for many years, it is quite a change to not see them anymore. As discussed above, even though it may sound cruel to keep staff out of the selling loop, it is actually best for all concerned. When you finally do sit down with employees to break the news, it's best to be upbeat and honest. Explain your reasons for the sale, if appropriate, and tell the staff that you have full confidence that they will do right by the new practice owner.

Thank them for their service and be sure to tell the new dentist, in front of the staff, that he's lucky to have such a talented and trustworthy group of individuals in his employ. Be prepared to answer their questions, as your employees will likely have many concerns about how new ownership will affect them. And be ready; emotions will arise and you'll need to handle them.

Second is closing the book on your practice and moving on. If you stick around the practice for a while to help staff and patients adjust, you'll find it difficult to "butt out" as the new owner puts his plans of operation into place. After all, it's been your baby all these years. You'll find yourself questioning his decisions and thinking, "This new guy doesn't know what he's doing. Why's he doing endo? I always referred it out." Or, "What's the big idea of using a payroll service? My wife always came in and did it." It's important that you move on. If you can't, then maybe you shouldn't have sold your practice.

Third, what are you going to do once you sell your practice? Having a plan in place prior to the sale is critically important. If you are one of the very few sellers who has truly thought out your future and has a master plan and the finances in place to embark on a new adventure or career, you'll do just fine. But, if you're like most, you will feel a void in your life for a while and have the desire or need to return to practice. It takes time to adjust to a new life, and it can be done, but if you want your future to be as happy as your career, you need to start planning.

The emotional considerations I've just laid out should be discussed with your broker, family, and financial advisors well before listing your practice for sale. Why you are selling and what kind of life you want to live and can afford to live must be decided prior to selling your practice. It may just make you change your mind before it's too late.

CASE STUDY **14**

Adjusting to the new dentist

One of my sellers had a terrible time letting go of his practice. "I'm worried about my staff," the doctor lamented to me a few months after the sale. As agreed in the contract, he had remained with the practice for a while to help the patients and staff adjust to the buyer. But when it came time to leave permanently, he was struggling. "I just don't like the way he handles the staff. He's too bossy." His comment sounded more like a concerned father than an employer.

I asked him to tell me what it was like when he bought the practice from the doctor who had built it. "Did you keep all the employees? Did you run the practice just like the seller did?"

"Oh, heck no," he told me emphatically. "We were two completely different types of people. He did his own endo and all his own hygiene. Can you imagine that? I referred the endo out and immediately hired a hygienist."

"And how did that work out?" I asked him.

"Just fine," he said adamantly "It took a little time, but eventually it worked out just fine." Then, he got kind of a funny look on his face, as if a lightbulb had come on in his head. "Hmmm, I think I see what you're getting at," he said calmly. "My staff will be okay. They'll have to adjust to the new boss just like they adjusted to me."

It can be difficult to watch another dentist take charge of your office and especially your employees. But you just have to let go and try to remember what it was like when you were the "new guy in town." The doctor let go and, somehow, the staff adjusted and did just fine.

17

How to Pass Employees Off to the Buyer after the Sale

Some of the material that follows is a repeat of Part 2. However, there is important material unique to the seller that should be read.

When you sell your dental practice, you not only leave your patients, you end the relationship you have had with your employees. The buyer becomes the employer. As mentioned earlier, this experience can trigger a bevy of emotions for you and staff members alike. And in addition, you have legal obligations to your employees that must be dealt with correctly to prevent potential violations of federal employment laws. Both buyer and seller must be protected during the transition period.

Some dentists are under the illusion that federal laws don't apply to them because they have very few employees. This is not the case. Federal employment laws apply to all businesses, regardless of size.

Let's look at how federal employment laws might affect transitioning staff members and the seller. Let's say that the seller had several employees who had been with the practice for varying periods of time. And let's assume that the employees want to keep their positions after the sale, which is the case 99 percent of the time. Normally, employees want and need their jobs. If the seller fails to terminate the staff members officially with a written notice and fails to get proofs of receipts of those notices, the seller could be liable for any errors the new employer (the buyer) makes. For example, let's say the buyer doesn't pay a staff member adequately for overtime. Without proper documentation of termination, the seller could be liable for the overtime pay along with any penalties and interest the labor board assesses.

Even worse, the labor board can review all documents pertaining to the case, as well as those of other employees, and their investigation can go back three years. The buyer, even though he had nothing to do with the employees prior to purchasing the practice, could be liable for any violations made by the seller in the past, along with penalties and interest. The amounts owed could be enormous. So, as you can see, both parties need to be protected during the practice sale.

In order to protect the buyer and the seller, both parties must take action. The buyer must interview each employee and rehire him or her individually (as an employee at will, of course). The seller must terminate each employee in writing and obtain proof of receipt from the employee. These two actions break the chain of employment and help protect both parties from employee law claims arising from the actions of their counterparts.

Also, make sure you pay each employee all their wages, overtime, and vacation pay *before* you quit the premises.

The labor board does not look favorably on employers who leave employees unpaid.

One last point about handling employees: We live in a litigious society, especially here in California. Your employees are being educated by attorneys on TV to "know their employee rights." They are being encouraged to take their employers to court if their federally mandated rights have been violated. You can't depend on ignorance of the labor laws to protect you. Your employees are getting smarter by the day. And trust me, there are employees out there who wouldn't hesitate to take their bosses to court if they felt they had suffered harm. This is another reason to work with an experienced and knowledgeable practice broker.

The letter you send to the patients

Once the sale of the practice has been finalized and the staff has been informed, a letter is sent out to all currently active patients. The letter I have used for years has been very well received. It thanks the patients for all their years of trust and introduces the new dentist and his or her qualifications. Both buyer and seller review the letter *before* it is printed on the seller's stationery, signed by the seller, and mailed.

CASE STUDY **15**

I thought my employees were friends and because of that, I thought they'd allow me to break the rules a bit.

Dr. B., like many dentists, thought his employees were his friends and because of that, he felt like he could bend the rules a bit. But he found out quickly, that isn't the case.

Dr. B. asked one of his employees if she could wait a week or so for her vacation pay. He was in the middle of changing banks and a little short on cash. "Oh, sure," was the employee's answer, until she got home and got her husband's input. He told her that the boss had to pay *all* the money she was owed when she signed her termination agreement. Whoops! Luckily, the employee called the doctor the minute she got home. The doctor asked her to come right back to the office and he paid her in full. That's what can happen if you don't follow the rules.

Remember, your employees are not your friends. They are employees and when it comes to disputes, the Employment Development Department always sides with the employees.

18

Tax Consequences of
Selling Your Practice

*T*he material that follows is a repeat of Part 2. It is included in case you are a seller and chose not to read Part 2 (Part 2 is about associates).

There can be substantial tax consequences for both parties in the sale of a dental practice. In general terms, the assets being sold in a dental practice include equipment, patient records, dental supplies, furniture, fixtures, goodwill, and covenant not to compete. The tax consequences have to do with how the various assets are allocated in the sale price. By changing the allocation value of the various assets, you can change the amount of tax that is owed.

Simply put, the seller's objective is usually to allocate the sale price of the assets to minimize the income tax owed on the gain. The buyer, on the other hand, would like to allocate the purchase price to accelerate the tax deduction on the assets. How the allocation is negotiated can have a significant bearing on the agreed-upon price. This is where a broker can really help. His negotiation skills, experience, and knowledge can make or break a deal. A conscientious, experienced, and principled broker will ensure that the purchase and sale of a dental practice is structured so that the process is a win-win situation for all concerned. Obviously, you'll want to meet with your CPA and attorney in *advance* of signing any documents to ensure that you are properly protected in the transaction. The importance of planning ahead cannot be overstated.

CASE STUDY **16**

I'm glad my CPA knew what he was doing

Dr. P. had purchased a practice from me twenty years ago and called me to say that he was selling his practice to his associate. He didn't want to use a broker and asked if it would be all right for him to just use the agreement that he had used when he bought the practice. I explained that there had been significant changes over the years and he should at least have a dental attorney and CPA review the document. He told me that his brother-in-law was an attorney and had already reviewed it. And he didn't have an accountant; he did his own tax returns. Despite my advice, Dr. P. didn't want to spend any money on professional advice.

I asked him to at least send me the page that listed the allocations of the purchase price. When he did and I looked at it, I was shocked. Almost all the allocation figures would be treated as ordinary income to the seller, and very little would be treated as capital gains. This helped the buyer only slightly, but killed the seller on taxes he would owe.

After consulting with my CPA, Alan Thomas, we readjusted the allocations more fairly for both buyer and seller. Dr. P. was thrilled with the end result. He saved $40,000 in taxes, while the buyer was barely affected at all. And the fees charged for that information were minimal.

19

Retirement

J've sold a lot of practices in the past twenty-five-plus years. I've seen many doctors succeed and some doctors fail in retirement. What I've learned is that how things turn out depends upon whether the dentist prepares adequately.

First and foremost, you need to have a plan. Having a plan in place *prior* to the sale is crucial. If you are one of the very fortunate sellers who has truly thought out your future and has a master plan and the finances in place to embark on a new adventure or career, you'll do just fine. It's been my experience that if dentists don't have something to *retire to* and expect to be *happy just because they are retiring,* they feel a void in their lives and have the desire or need to return to practice.

Just like when you have a new baby in the house, or get married or divorced, it takes time to adjust to a new life. You'll have challenges adjusting to so much time on your hands. But it can be done.

I recommend that clients have multiple discussions with their brokers, family members, and financial advisors *well* in advance of listing their practices for sale. Selling a dental practice requires specialized knowledge and the support of skilled professionals to achieve your goals with the least possible risk. Why you are selling and what kind of life you want to live and can afford to live must be decided prior to selling your practice. In some cases, it may just make you change your mind before it's too late.

About a written retirement plan Your written plan *does not* have to be developed by an expensive estate planner. In most cases, estate planning services are about selling life insurance. What you need is a written plan that contains a list of all of your projected income sources and projected living expenses after you retire. (Get help from your CPA if you are unsure how to calculate income from pension plans, 401Ks, etc.)

In the Appendices, you'll find two documents that can be used to develop your retirement plan: *Estimated Income Analysis* and *Estimated Expenses in Retirement*. Invest the time to fill out these forms completely and accurately. Be realistic and add at least 10 percent inflation each year. When they are complete, you'll have a good idea if you can afford the life you want during retirement.

CASE STUDY **17**

Please . . . somebody stop me!

"What are you going to do, Dr. J., when you retire?" I always ask that question when I'm discussing the sale of a practice. About twelve years ago, I sold a very nice practice in Cypress. The doctor gave me all the right answers as to why he was selling: he had plenty of money to retire, he wanted to start an antique business in which he and his wife could work together, and he was ready to move on. I was able to sell his practice and he was very appreciative of the job I had done.

A couple of years later, Dr. J. called me with some unhappy news. He had lost a lot of money in real estate and the stock market, and although he loved his antiquing business, it wasn't making the kind of money he had expected. He wanted, no, **needed**, to find a dental practice. We found him a practice and he worked another four years, after which he retired again. But this time, with the money he earned, he made safer, more conservative investments. Also, the real estate market and stock market rebounded.

I am happy to report that Dr. J. is now financially sound. The moral of the story is be sure that you have enough money to retire **before** you take that important step. And don't make those determinations alone; consult a professional. A little money spent up front can prevent a lot of misery on the back end.

20

How to choose a practice broker

This information is repeated from Part 2. It is included in case you are a seller and chose not to read Part 2.

No two dentists are alike, and so it is with dental brokers. When choosing a dental practice broker look for experience, integrity, and proven expertise in the industry. Most dental practice brokers hire salespeople to answer the phone. This can be frustrating and a colossal waste of time, having to explain the same stuff to a different person each time you call the broker's office. Ask with whom you'll be speaking when you call the office. If your contact person changes with the weather, find another broker. Look for a broker with banking contacts, dental attorney contacts, and CPA connections. Be sure your broker has a working knowledge of how a dental office operates and understands the difference between a fee-for-service office and managed care office. It's critically important to sell your practice to a buyer that not only fits his needs, but fits his skills and temperament as well. When you sell your practice to the right buyer, it is better for the patients and staff. The buyer will enjoy dentistry more, and that usually equates to a more beneficial situation for all concerned.

A retired dentist makes a better broker.

I believe that being a dentist gives me special insights that a non-dentist broker doesn't have. Most brokers aren't dentists. They don't know the difference between one practice and another. Being a dentist, I do. Also, because I'm a dentist, I understand how to read patient charts. Oftentimes I can see incomplete dentistry in those charts that a new dentist might be able to tap. Or I see in the charts that the selling doctor has very little dentistry left to be completed. Being able to read patient charts is an asset that non-dental brokers lack.

Also, I understand overhead and know what the norms should be. Practice numbers tell a story if the reader knows the language. Because I practiced dentistry for over fifteen years, I'm savvy to what the numbers say. This is really helpful with matching buyers and sellers. And it's incredibly important when dealing with banks who will loan money to the buyers. I know how new patient flow fits into the picture as well. In addition, in-depth knowledge of practice management can be a powerful negotiating tool. Plus, my dental experience helps me see and understand the *kind* of practice I am trying to sell. Knowing whether the buyer is a good fit for the practice I have listed can be extremely beneficial. For example, if the buyer wants a low-key practice seeing only a few patients a day, he or she would be miserable in a fast-paced environment that sees twenty patients a day.

In short, as a retired dentist I know the important questions to ask. And I know what the answers to those questions say about the practice I am selling. For example: What kind of procedures does the seller do? Does he do endo? Does he place implants? Does he do ortho? Does he do his own hygiene, or does he have a hygienist? And, as I've said before, how many patients a day does he see? These are vital considerations when trying to match a buyer and seller.

CASE STUDY **18**

Why I became a practice sales broker

The reason I became a practice sales broker was because of my desire to help my peers. And the reason I thought my fellow dentists needed help was because of the experiences I had when selling my practice. When I sold my practice in 1992, I interviewed two different brokers, both of whom were well known. They both told me I could get a very high selling price, higher than I expected. Alan Thomas, my accountant, warned me that he didn't think that price was reasonable. But I fell for the bait. I should have listed to Alan.

Months passed without an offer, and finally when I started getting offers they were significantly lower than the listing. Not a few thousand less, but tens of thousands less. The broker I had picked told me that I should take the offer and that he hadn't guaranteed the price we had agreed upon. I felt betrayed and lied to. The broker made me feel like an idiot and like my best interests were not being considered. He wanted his commission.

That experience influences how we treat our clients. Today, when I take a listing, I **put in writing** that if I can't get the price at which I appraised the practice, then the seller has no obligation whatsoever to accept the offer. The choice is solely the seller's. I never force anyone to sell. And I never make a seller feel like an idiot. I try very hard to educate the seller before taking the listing and during the entire process.

Appendices

Overhead Analysis Templates

How does your overhead compare? Are you unsure what the optimum percentages should be for each item in your dental practice overhead? Don't be. The following **Over-head Analysis Templates** were compiled by Thomas & Fees Accountancy Corp. and based on practice data collected *over four decades of experience working primarily with dentists*. They can be used to compare your practice numbers to the norm.

Please Note: Expense percentages differ according to the type of practice being analyzed. These templates are for the most common dental practices. To download templates for free, visit our website http://tfpsales.com.

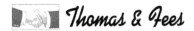
Thomas & Fees

Overhead Analysis Template
PRACTICE WITH SOLO DENTIST
Appendix A

Office of:_____

Month of: _____

	PERCENTAGE		AMOUNT	
STATEMENT OF INCOME	Optimum	Actual	Current Month	Year to Date
Accounts Receivable				
Production	100%			
Collections	95% - 98%			
Expenses				
Salaries - Hygienist	5% - 9%			
Salaries - Staff	14% - 17%			
Payroll Taxes	2%			
Lab	8%			
Professional Supplies	6%			
Rent & Utilities	8%			
Office Supplies & Computer	3%			
Legal, Accounting & Collection	2%			
Telephone	1%			
Insurance	2%			
Group Ins. & Employee Benefits	2%			
Advertising	1%			
Other Business Expenses	4%			
Maintenance				
Promotion				
Education & Seminars				
Dues & Subscriptions				
Equipment Rental				
Licenses & Permits				
TOTAL EXPENSE	60%			
NET CASH INCOME	40%	%	$	$

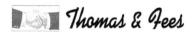

Overhead Analysis Template
PRACTICE WITH ASSOCIATES
Appendix B

Office of:_____

Month of: _____

STATEMENT OF INCOME	PERCENTAGE		AMOUNT	
	Optimum	Actual	Current Month	Year to Date
Accounts Receivable				
Production	100%			
Collections	95% - 98%			
Expenses				
Salaries - Associate	5% - 10%			
Salaries - Hygienist	5% - 9%			
Salaries - Staff	14% - 17%			
Payroll Taxes	3%			
Lab	8%			
Professional Supplies	6%			
Rent & Utilities	4%			
Office Supplies & Computer	3%			
Legal, Accounting & Collection	1%			
Telephone	1%			
Insurance	2%			
Group Ins. & Employee Benefits	2%			
Advertising	1%			
Other Business Expenses	8%			
Maintenance				
Promotion				
Education & Seminars				
Dues & Subscriptions				
Equipment Rental				
Licenses & Permits				
TOTAL EXPENSE	70%			
NET CASH INCOME	30%	%	$	$

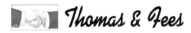 *Thomas & Fees*

Overhead Analysis Template
ORTHODONTICS PRACTICE
Appendix C

Office of:_____

Month of: _____

STATEMENT OF INCOME	PERCENTAGE		AMOUNT	
	Optimum	Actual	Current Month	Year to Date
Collections	100%			
Expenses				
Salaries - Staff	17% - 22%			
Payroll Taxes	2%			
Lab	1% - 3%			
Professional Supplies	6% - 9%			
Rent & Utilities	5%			
Office Supplies & Computer	3%			
Legal, Accounting & Collection	1%			
Telephone	1%			
Insurance	2%			
Group Ins. & Employee Benefits	2%			
Advertising	1%			
Other Business Expenses	4%			
Maintenance				
Promotion				
Education & Seminars				
Dues & Subscriptions				
Equipment Rental				
Licenses & Permits				
TOTAL EXPENSE	50%			
NET CASH INCOME	50%	%	$	$

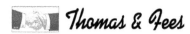
Thomas & Fees

Overhead Analysis Template
ORAL SURGERY PRACTICE
Appendix D

Office of:_____

Month of: _____

STATEMENT OF INCOME	PERCENTAGE		AMOUNT	
	Optimum	Actual	Current Month	Year to Date
Accounts Receivable		_____	_____	_____
Production	100%	_____	_____	_____
Collections	98%	_____	_____	_____
Expenses		_____	_____	_____
Salaries - Staff	14% - 20%	_____	_____	_____
Payroll Taxes	3%	_____	_____	_____
Professional Supplies	8%	_____	_____	_____
Rent & Utilities	8%	_____	_____	_____
Office Supplies & Computer	3%	_____	_____	_____
Legal, Accounting & Collection	2%	_____	_____	_____
Telephone	1%	_____	_____	_____
Insurance	2%	_____	_____	_____
Group Ins. & Employee Benefits	2%	_____	_____	_____
Advertising	1%	_____	_____	_____
Other Business Expenses	4%	_____	_____	_____
Maintenance				
Promotion				
Education & Seminars				
Dues & Subscriptions				
Equipment Rental				
Licenses & Permits				
TOTAL EXPENSE	50%	_____	_____	_____
NET CASH INCOME	50%	_____ %	$ _____	$ _____

Retirement Analysis Templates

Can you afford to retire? Use these templates to determine if you can.

Thomas & Fees

Overhead Analysis Template
ESTIMATED INCOME ANALYSIS
Appendix E

Office of:_____
Month of: _____

	Per Month	Per Year (x12)		Net After Taxes
Tax-Free Bonds			x 1 =	
Interest Income			x .67 =	
Dividends (stocks, etc.)			x .67 =	
* Social Security Benefits			x 1 =	
** Pension Payouts			x .67 =	
			TOTAL	

* Social Security Benefits

  – Check with your accountant to determine when to take your Social Security and
    how much would be taxable.
  – Social Security benefits are limited between ages 62 and 66, based upon your other
    income.

** Pension Payouts

  – Can start at age 59½
  – Must start taking out at age 70½
  – Average payout is 5% of fund balance/year.

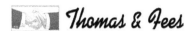

Thomas & Fees

Overhead Analysis Template
ESTIMATED EXPENSES IN RETIREMENT
Appendix F

Directions: Will your income in retirement meet your spending needs? Use this template to estimate your monthly expenses in retirement. Accuracy counts. Your lifestyle will be diminished if your figures are wrong. The most commonly missed items are real estate taxes, insurance premiums, medical expenses, and home and auto repairs. Add 10 percent for cost of living increases over time.

	Month 1	Month 2	Month 3	Average	Year
Morgage or Rent					
Property Taxes					
Homeowners Insurance					
Utilities					
Maintenance/Fees					
Food					
Dining Out					
Transportation					
Vehicle Maintenance					
Fuel					
Auto Insurance					
Medical Services					
Medications & Supplies					
Health Insurance					
Life Insurance					
Longterm Care Insurance					
Other Insurance					
Clothing					
Alimony					
Loans/Credit Cards					
Travel/Vacation					
Entertainment					
Hobbies					
Gifts					
Charitable Contributions					
Other					
Total Monthly Expences					

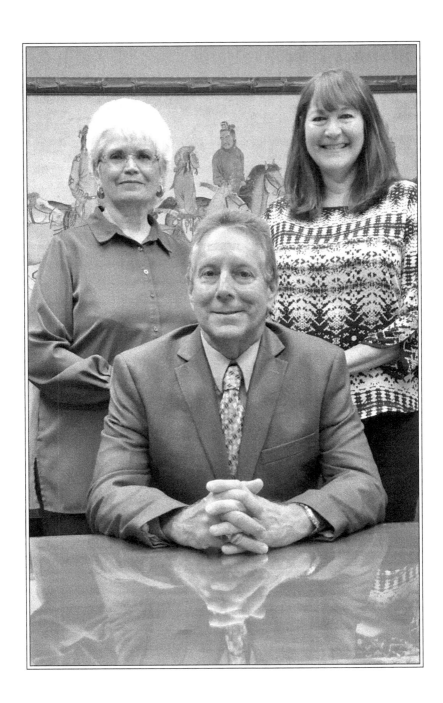

About the Author

and Thomas & Fees Practice Sales

Our Broker Is a Retired Dentist – Most practice sales firms hire salesmen to sell practices. And, while they may be competent in the technical end of practice sales, they know nothing about dentistry. Because our broker is a successful, retired dentist, he has unique insights into the career of a dentist. He understands the concerns facing a dentist in his or her first job as an associate. From the dentist's first job to the purchase of the first practice, right down to the sale of the practice and retirement, Dr. Kempler has done it all.

Dr. Philip L. Kempler – Graduated from Cornell University in 1974 and the University of Pennsylvania Dental School in 1978. He did his residency at the V.A. Hospital at Wadsworth in Los Angeles, and retired after owning a highly successful dental practice for fifteen years. Driven by the desire to help his peers traverse the challenges of building successful careers in dentistry, he became a broker in 1993.

Reputation and Experience – We have over twenty-five years' experience and a proven track record for honest, fair, and reliable business practices.

Our Parent Company is Thomas & Fees Accountancy Corporation

Experience – Thomas & Fees Accountancy Corp. has been working primarily with dentists for *over four decades.* During that time, we have guided hundreds of young dentists through their careers. We've helped them navigate successfully into their first associate positions and, when the time was right, helped them maneuver through the complexities of practice purchase. For the buyer, the oldest CPA firm in California working primarily with dentists is sure to have a continuing supply of exceptional practices for sale. And when it's time to sell, with over six hundred dental clients, sellers can rest assured that their practices will be exposed to a ready list of qualified buyers.

We Understand Dentists – Decades of dental contacts means you won't be advised by a professional who has to guess or experiment. Deciding when it's the right time to sell, both emotionally and financially, and making that important career decision to purchase a practice, shouldn't be decided by beginners or part-time sales associates.

We Have a Long-term Relationship – Having ongoing and multifaceted relationships with clients guarantees that decisions aren't driven by commissions.

Reputation – You can't stay in business serving dentists for forty-plus years without high integrity, proven knowledge, and unique dental know-how. Proudly, Thomas & Fees Accountancy Corp. has a reputation that is envied in

the industry. Their motto says it all: "We want to be partners in your financial success."

Thomas & Fees Practice Sales

511 E. First St., Suite C

Tustin, CA 92780

Office: (714) 544-4341 Home Office: (949) 362-4749

http://tfpsales.com

CPSIA information can be obtained
at www.ICGtesting.com
Printed in the USA
FSHW020443150119

9 780999 473030